Let's Get Started

First of all, thank you for purchasing this book.

I would like to remind you that the beginning is halfway to finish.

You're great!

Now take a deep breath.

Please stand up.

Go infront of the mirror.

And take a picture.

I'm gonna tell you why I want you to take pictures in the last chapter of the book.

About the Author

I was born in 1993 in Swindon. After completing my primary and my high school education in 2011, I started the University of Bradford Healthcare Sciences in the UK.

I graduated from there in 2015. During this period, I completed my seminar on Min Minerals in Cancer and my thesis on Etk The Effect of Treatment Method in Cancer Disease on Nutrition thesis.

As soon as I graduated, I started my internship at Glenfield General Hospital. Then I moved to Bedford Hospital in 2016, where I continued to work as a dietician.

During this period, I decided to continue my education and I started to educate at the university I graduated from.

What Will You Learn ?

In this book you will first learn what to do to eat healthy.

But it won't stop there.

You will also learn how to maintain a healthy form and even lose weight while eating healthy.

Of course, I will be sharing a very ambitious program with you.

Who Is This Book For ?

This book is my favorite question for whom I guess the question.

This is the book for those who will not get bored of applying the information written inside.

This is the book for those who will make this information a goal and never give up.

This is the book for those who call it from wherever the damage returns.

This book is the book that you won't give up if you fail in the first application.

This is the book for those who believe in this information.

You will succeed if you don't stop believing! If not today, then tomorrow!
The results will stay the same!

Who Is This Book Not For ?

This book is not intended for people who do not believe in healthy eating.

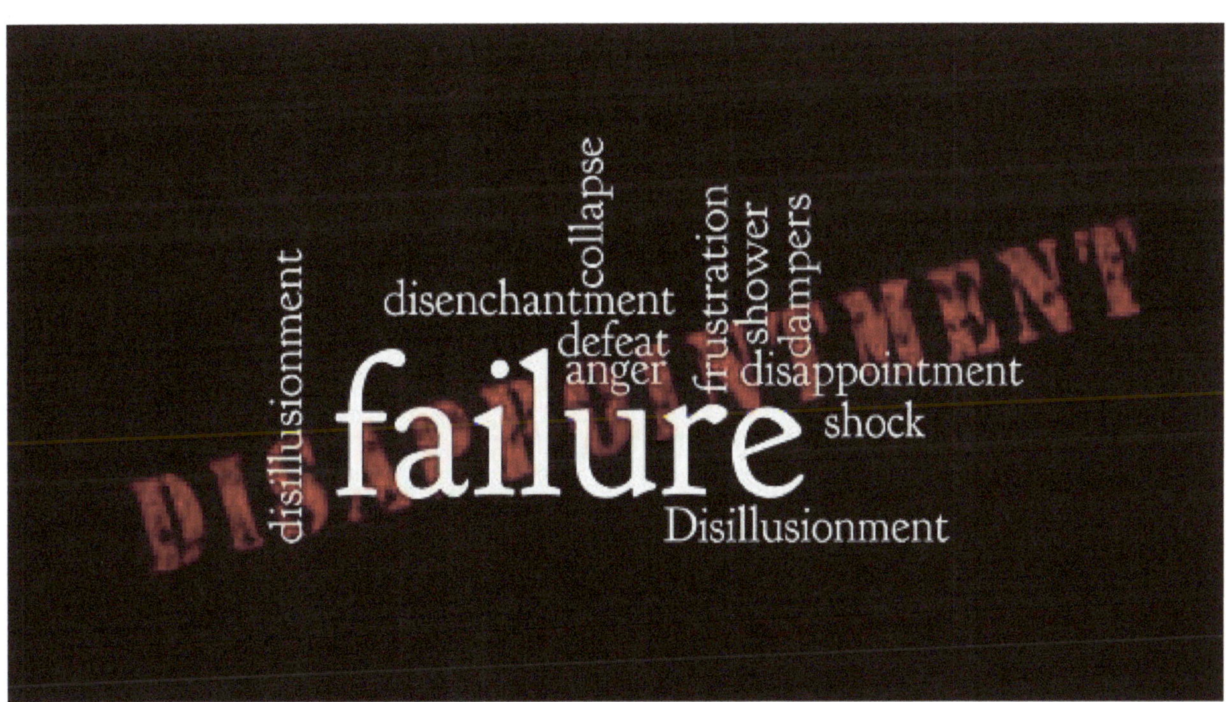

Purpose Of The Book

The first purpose of this book is to show you the basics of a healthy life, its philosophy.

Once you understand the philosophy of this issue, you need to integrate it into your life.

And in this direction, you need to train yourself and run towards this goal.

What I can do to show you at this point is limited. The rest will unveil itself with your faith.

My Opinion

Before I share this book with you, I applied every word written here to my own life.

Of course, I have a healthy life as a result of the school I studied, the way I work and the way I am used to.

But every word here has a lot to do with my life.

Think about it, how much will this affect a life of someone who is not healthy.

To succeed, you must first dream.

You should ask later.

And you have to fight without losing faith.

Content

Healthy Nutrition

List to Lose Weight

Fast and Feel Great

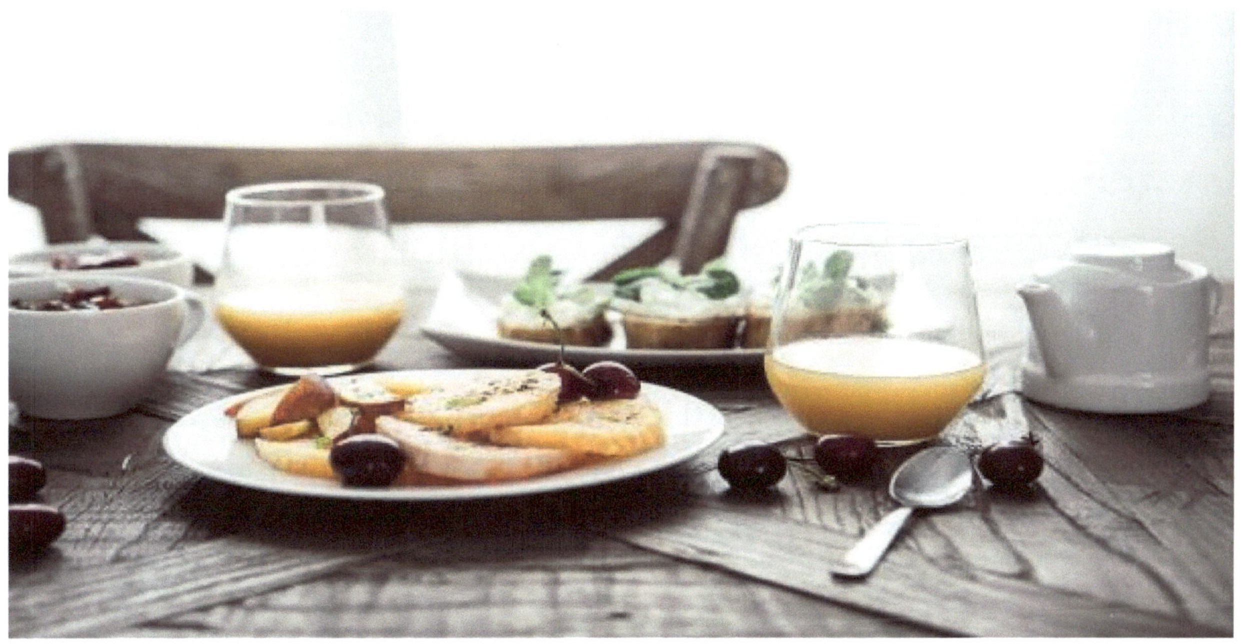

Introduction

This article we prepared about healthy nutrition is not based on prejudice or ethics, but based on scientific research results.

Healthy eating, healthy living, being fit and staying fit. All these concepts are linked in a cause and effect relationship. When you remove one or more of the chains, the whole balance is disrupted. In this article, we will share nutritional recommendations based on high nutritional and low carbohydrate foods. We can call this nutrition list a hid low carb, nutritious, real food based besleme feed list.

What is nutritious, low carb food?

Low-carbohydrate nutrition minimizes sugar and starch, replacing them with foods rich in protein and healthy fats.

"Real food" means choosing food that humans have access to throughout evolution. Non-natural foods processed with artificial chemicals are avoided.

The low carbohydrate nutrition program is not a "program abil that can be applied for a while. A lifestyle change is a diet.

It is a healthy diet based on the food that people have consumed for hundreds of thousands of years before the agricultural and industrial revolutions.

Low-carbohydrate nutrition has been shown to be much more effective than the recommended low-fat diet around the world.

What should not be eaten in a healthy nutrition program?

Foods that should be limited in healthy eating lists are;

Sugar: Extra sugar addiction, obesity and obesity are the leading causes of diabetes and cardiovascular diseases.

Cereals: If you want to lose weight, you need to avoid all cereals, including bread and pasta. Gluten grains (wheat, barley and rye) are the worst. If you are not trying to lose weight, you can consume healthy cereals such as rice and oats.

Seed and vegetable oils: Soybean oil, corn oil and others. These are processed harmful fats that contain large amounts of Omega-6 fatty acids.

Trans fats: Genetically modified fats that are very harmful to health. It is usually found in processed foods.

<u>Artificial sweeteners:</u> Although calorie-free, studies show that it is associated with obesity and related diseases. Choose Stevia if you need to use a sweetener.

<u>Iyet Diet "and" low-fat "products:</u> Most of these" healthy foods ir are not healthy at all. These products containing artificial sweeteners are as bad as agave syrup sugar.

<u>Processed foods:</u> Highly processed foods are generally low in nutrients. Contains high levels of unhealthy and unnatural chemicals.

You should read the contents before you consume packaged products, you will not believe the amount of harmful food contained in it.

What Are Healthy Foods?

You should eat natural, unprocessed food that people are genetically adapted to. Research shows that this type of food is great in terms of health.

For healthy people who do not need to lose weight, there is absolutely no proven reason to prevent tubers such as potatoes and sweet potatoes, and healthier gluten-free cereals such as oats and rice.

If you are overweight or have problems with metabolism (low HDL, high LDL cholesterol, triglycerides, regional fat, etc.), you should restrict all foods containing high amounts of carbohydrates.

Which Foods Should Be on the Healthy Nutrition List?

<u>Meat:</u> Beef, lamb, pork, chicken and so on. People have eaten meat for hundreds of thousands of years. Raw meat of animals fed with natural feed is one of the best protein sources.

<u>Fish:</u> Fish is great. It is very healthy, satisfying and rich in omega-3 fatty acids and other nutrients. You should eat fish every week (preferably salmon).

<u>Eggs:</u> Eggs are among the most nutritious foods on the planet. Yolk is the most nutritious and healthy part. Egg feeder is a source of omega3.

<u>Vegetables:</u> It contains fiber and many nutrients required for human body. Vegetables should be consumed every day.

<u>Fruit:</u> It is rich in fiber and vitamin C. It is high in sugar. If you are trying to lose weight, you should take care to consume it in a moderate way.

<u>Nuts and seeds:</u> Almond, walnut, sunflower seeds and so on. In terms of vitamins and minerals, the calories of nuts are very high. If you are trying to lose weight, you should consume it carefully.

<u>Potato:</u> Root vegetables such as potatoes and sweet potatoes are high carbohydrate foods. If you need to lose weight you should consume.

<u>High-fat dairy products:</u> Cheese, cream, butter, whole-fat yogurt, etc. These foods are rich in healthy fats and calcium. Milk obtained from grass-fed cows is rich in vitamin K2, which is very important for health.

<u>Fats and oils:</u> Olive oil, butter, sunflower oil and so on. When frying, prefer more saturated oils.

Drink Tips for Healthy Living

- **<u>Coffee:</u>** Coffee is very rich in antioxidants, but people who are sensitive to caffeine should be careful about coffee consumption. Don't drink coffee late in the day because you can ruin your sleep.

- **<u>Tea:</u>** Tea is healthy, rich in antioxidants and contains much less caffeine than coffee.

- **<u>Water:</u>** Drink plenty of water throughout the day and especially during and after exercise.

- **<u>Mineral water:</u>** Mineral soda without artificial sweeteners is healthy.

Avoid all beverages containing sugar and artificial sweeteners. Alcohol and fruit juices are also very sugary and calorie.

A simple rule; do not consume calorie drinks.

Foods to be consumed in a moderate way

- **Dark Chocolate:** Prefer 70% more cocoa organic chocolate. Dark chocolate is rich in healthy fats and antioxidants.

- **Alcohol:** Choose wines and beverages without extra sugar or carbohydrates: vodka, whiskey, etc.

What is the Daily Carbohydrate Amount in Healthy Nutrition Lists?

The amount of carbohydrate per day varies according to gender, age and person.

However, you can consider the following amounts as a general guide:

<u>10-20 grams per day:</u> means that no carbohydrate is consumed except for very low, low carb vegetables. It may be appropriate for those with metabolic problems, those trying to lose weight and those with diabetes.

<u>If you need to gain weight quickly:</u> 20-50 grams per day. You can consume a few servings of fruit and vegetables a day.

<u>This is the most accurate amount:</u> 50-150 grams per day. Fruits, vegetables and even some starch sources for healthy living help you capture this amount daily.

When you reduce your carbohydrate intake to less than 50 grams a day, you can't eat any sugar, bread, pasta, cereal, potatoes and more than 1 fruit per day.

<u>**Warning for diabetic patients:**</u> Carbohydrates on the nutritional list are broken down into glucose in the digestive tract and then enter the body as blood sugar. If you eat less carbohydrates, you will need less insulin and glucose-lowering medications.

It is very dangerous for your blood sugar to fall below a certain level (hypoglycemia). If you have diabetes, consult your doctor before reducing carbohydrate intake

A Healthy Nutrition List That Can Save Lives

This is an exemplary diet plan that contains less than 50 grams of carbohydrates per day for a week.

Day 1 - Monday:

Breakfast: Omelette with various vegetables, made from butter or coconut oil.

Lunch: Yogurt with blueberries and a handful of almonds.

Dinner: Cheeseburger (without bread), served with vegetables and salsa sauce.

Day 2 - Tuesday:

Breakfast: Bacon and eggs.

Lunch: Burgers and vegetables from the previous evening.

Dinner: Boiled salmon with butter and vegetables.

Day 3 - Wednesday:

Breakfast: Eggs and vegetables in butter or coconut oil.

Lunch: Shrimp salad with some olive oil.

Dinner: Grilled chicken with vegetables.

Day 4 - Thursday:

Breakfast: Omelette with vegetables, butter or coconut oil.

Lunch: Smoothie prepared with coconut milk, fruit, almond and protein powder.

Dinner: Steak and vegetables.

Day 5 - Friday:

Breakfast: Bacon and Eggs.

Lunch: Chicken salad with little olive oil.

Dinner: Chops with vegetables.

Day 6 - Saturday:

Breakfast: Omelette with vegetables.

Lunch: Herbal yogurt with strawberries, coconut and a handful of walnuts.

Dinner: Meatballs with vegetables.

Day 7 - Sunday:

Breakfast: Bacon and Eggs.

Lunch: Coconut milk, some cream, chocolate flavored protein powder and fruit.

Dinner: Grilled chicken wings with some raw spinach.

Healthy diet lists are rich in vegetables. If you want to stay under 50 grams of carbohydrate per day, then you can eat a small portion of fruit or some strawberries every day.

The meat of animals fed with organic and natural herbs is the best. If you can find them, add them to your nutrition list.

What Are Healthy Snacks?

There is no scientific evidence that you should not eat 3 meals a day. If you get hungry between meals, you can see healthy snacks below.

- **Full fat yogurt**

- **One serving of fruit**

- **Baby carrots**

- **Very boiled eggs**

- **A handful of nuts**

- **Some cheese and meat**

Result

The list of healthy diets can be made monthly, weekly or several weeks.

This list, which must be prepared by a qualified
dietitian, is prepared individually.

You need a balanced diet to get a certain amount of everything the body needs.

Thus, you will have a healthy life and stay fit and fit.

References

https://www.ncbi.nlm.nih.gov/pmc/articles/PMC2673878/

https://www.ncbi.nlm.nih.gov/pmc/articles/PMC2235907/

https://care.diabetesjournals.org/content/33/11/2477.short

https://www.ncbi.nlm.nih.gov/pubmed/17921363

https://www.ncbi.nlm.nih.gov/pmc/articles/PMC1954879/

https://www.ncbi.nlm.nih.gov/pubmed/21224837

https://www.ncbi.nlm.nih.gov/pubmed/6111631

https://www.ncbi.nlm.nih.gov/pubmed/12145006

https://www.ncbi.nlm.nih.gov/pubmed/17206762

https://www.ncbi.nlm.nih.gov/pubmed/21118617

https://www.ncbi.nlm.nih.gov/pubmed/17700650

https://academic.oup.com/jn/article/135/3/562/4663700

https://www.ncbi.nlm.nih.gov/pubmed/9322581

https://www.ncbi.nlm.nih.gov/pubmed/18535548

https://care.diabetesjournals.org/content/32/4/688.short

https://www.ncbi.nlm.nih.gov/pubmed/17583796

https://www.ncbi.nlm.nih.gov/pubmed/19209185

https://www.ncbi.nlm.nih.gov/pubmed/17522610

https://www.ncbi.nlm.nih.gov/pubmed/17684196

Final Words

We came to an end.

I applaud you for coming so far and not giving up.

You're great.

When you look in the mirror again, you will understand how this first week of one week passed.

Don't worry if you're on your way to losing weight, and you don't get any results in the first period. You have to continue.

If the goal is to transition to a healthy diet, you should have already seen the differences in your body. Even if you can't, I can. From the very beginning, your skin is shining!

You're great!

Note

Save your first and last photo :)

And don't hesitate to contact me when you want to ask something that you have in mind, or when you have something to share.

Contact info : dr.davidfisher.nutritionist@gmail.com